DRUG TESTING AND THE WORKPLACE

DRUG TESTING AND THE WORKPLACE

Jim Kelaher, MD, MPH, CPA

To order additional copies of this book, contact:
Xlibris Corporation
1-888-795-4274
www.Xlibris.com
Orders@Xlibris.com
23332

CONTENTS

FOREWARD

Drug testing is playing an increasingly important role in the hiring process and during employment. Therefore, it is increasingly important that human resource personnel and others have a good understanding of drug testing programs. Further, an increasing number of health care professionals are becoming involved in testing. As a physician, my experience relates to medical aspects of drug use. However, as an occupational physician that experience also relates to administrative and human resource issues within drug testing.

Drug Testing and the Workplace gives the reader important, practical information about developing and running drug testing programs. Whether you are new to drug testing and need a good foundation or have experience with it and are interested in supplemental information, this book should serve as a resource.

INTRODUCTION

Drug Testing

Employee drug testing certainly is not new. It is gaining more and more acceptance in the workplace. In fact, many companies pride themselves on their efforts to deter drug use in the workplace. Walk into many retail establishments and you will see a prominently displayed sign reading: "If you use drugs, don't apply here." Nonetheless, it can remain a source of headaches for anyone who tries to start a program, or worse, who has to deal with some of the test results.

However, once set up, a drug testing program should not be very burdensome. A program is for the employees' benefit as well. People do not want to work next to someone who is under the influence. In general, employees will accept such a program, but the employer has an obligation to run a program that is fair and accurate. Inaccurate results can end up inadvertently discriminating against employees/applicants. It can result in mistrust and even formal complaints. This, of course, should not happen. Naturally, a poorly run program cannot accomplish its goal.

The following sections describe the nuts and bolts of setting up and running an employment drug testing program. In addition, the sections provide a lot of the rationale behind common practices. Although this is more than most readers will need, it helps to illustrate that some things are not purely random or for no reason. On the other hand, some practices provide the employer with a lot of discretion. This is important so that you can adapt a program to fit *your* needs. Nonetheless, no book can act as a guarantee that reading it cover to cover will allow you to have the perfect program. This book alone will not be enough for you to completely set up and run your program.

In medicine, in order to interpret any test like a blood test or even an x-ray, we have to ask ourselves why we are doing the test. Although a test result may be fairly objective, its significance can vary substantially depending on what the practitioner was expecting to find. We may be looking to screen for abnormal conditions, confirm a specific diagnosis, or conduct follow-up for treatment. The same is true with an employment drug test. Certain findings may not be unexpected and others may be ambiguous. There has to be some understanding of what a test does and does not accomplish.

The basic premise of drug testing is that using (illegal) drugs does impair performance. Impaired performance can cause accidents and endanger others. In the late 80's there were several events which gained a lot of public attention. This included the well known event of the *Exxon Valdez*, the oil tanker which went ashore in Alaska. The National Transportation Safety Board cited several factors contributing to the cause of the accident. These included "possible impairment from alcohol." The captain was actually found not guilty of operating a vessel while under the influence of alcohol, but the role of alcohol remained a large focus of the investigation.

The Federal government implemented laws *requiring* drug testing of certain groups of employees in the transportation industry. This was not necessarily the beginning of drug testing in the workplace, but it usually serves as a starting point in most people's minds.

OK, so you don't have a lot of tanker captains working in your office supply shop. Does this mean that the Government says you have to do drug testing? Probably not. Does it mean that you can't? Of course not. SAMHSA, Substance Abuse and Mental Health Services Administration, estimates that over 7% of full-time workers report current, illicit drug use. A similar number are described as heavy alcohol users. This information comes from the National Household Survey on Drug Abuse, 1997. In that survey, employees also reported that about 49% of employers had some type of drug testing program. So, if it is not required, but you are allowed to do testing, should you? Before you decide, look at some of the issues surrounding a drug testing program.

DECIDING TO HAVE A DRUG TESTING PROGRAM

Required Testing

As mentioned before, the Federal government requires testing of certain transportation industry employees. Most people in this line of business are well aware of their obligations. So, if you are unaware of this, you probably are not in that group. The U.S. Department of Transportation (DOT) developed laws that requires testing of employees who have safety-sensitive job duties in the transportation industry. Note that these rules require private sector employers to implement their own drug testing programs; the Federal government does not do the testing or select employees for testing. The government makes the rules and has an enforcement function. The transportation employees who are covered include truck drivers, airline pilots (and mechanics), people who work on ships, train conductors and even pipeline workers. Safety-sensitive basically means those whose lack of job performance could pose a danger to the public. Incidentally, DOT does require alcohol testing as well. Obviously, a truck driver who cannot maintain good control of his/her truck can endanger others. The full scope of who is covered is not very relevant here, but some points are. First, not everybody who drives as part of their job has to be tested. The DOT requires testing of those who are required to have a commercial driver's license (CDL). Likewise, the DOT defines which employees in the air, rail and sea industries need to be tested. Next, the DOT is not the only agency that has laws governing drug testing. The Department of Energy has also set forth rules for testing workers.

The *Drug Free Workplace Act* (public law 100-71, Executive Order 12564) also imposes some requirements on employers. DFWA covers all entities that receive federal funding in excess of $25,000. However, unlike the DOT, it does not mandate drug testing. Rather, it requires employers to: have a policy about drug testing, educate employees about that policy, and educate employees about the adverse affect of drugs. In Texas, there are requirements from the Texas Worker's Compensation Commission that subscribers with more than 15 employees must have a policy regarding drug abuse (Sec. 411.091). Many cities require its contractors to not only have a drug policy but to do some sort of random drug testing. The requirements tend not to be very specific.

While I am not entirely familiar with requirements in other places, I am fairly confident to assert that many localities have similar requirements. As you can see there is not only a variety in the regulatory bodies that can (and do) impose rules, but the extent of obligation imposed and the level of detail provided varies substantially.

If you are looking for the one source that tells you everything you need to know about who is covered and how to do it, it ain't out there. But, in practice, the best approach is to ask people who do this regularly. That may include colleagues in the same profession or people who make a living doing drug testing. Even this is not a guarantee, since no one can know every possible rule out there. Required elements, if any, will vary. Of those I have seen, the DOT rules are the most detailed. Clearly, no one can give your business a certificate or whatever indicating that you are in total compliance. One agency that does not regulate drug testing is the Occupational Safety and Health Administration (OSHA). A diligent search, however, should reveal whether you are regulated. Any business that does business with a governmental entity, whether local, state or federal, should review the process for bidding and the rules for doing business with that entity to ensure compliance. Obviously, these rules cover issues like fiscal responsibilities, records, and insurance requirements, but would usually mention drug testing requirements.

Where to check for more information about required testing:

- Federal Agencies

Particularly those that regulate your line of business. They may have requirements in order for you to receive funding or to submit bids.

- State Agencies

Industry or labor board

- Trade associations

Many associations have member services that can be helpful. Their publications may also be useful.

- Worker's compensation insurer

They have a vested interest in your company's safety

Should I Do Drug Testing?

Again, this is a personal choice. Certainly, a legal mandate is a good reason to do something. Far and away most employers do not fall under a mandated program. However, drug testing is becoming more popular. Many companies actually use it as a competitive edge. This occurs on the consumer level and within industry "benchmarking." I do not have an elaborate, in-depth treatise on this point. Basically, the consensus in society is (probably) that using drugs is wrong. Taking a stance against drug use is good. So, it may give consumers a warm, fuzzy feeling knowing that they deal with the "good guys." Companies may boast about rainforest safe furniture, recycled products, dolphin-free tuna, and now drug testing. On the industry level, vendors may look for this when putting out bids, insurers may look favorably at it, and it is just seen as a good practice within the safety industry.

In theory, it should save money. If we can reduce or eliminate drug use, we should reduce accidents, which should save money. In some states, proof of drug/alcohol use can be used to deny a worker's compensation claim. It is hard to say how accurate some estimates are in calculating the amount saved by doing drug testing. For one thing, many programs are implemented as part of larger safety programs so attributing savings to drug testing just cannot be allocated. Additionally, you would ideally need to know your accident rates and costs due to drug use. To do this, you need to compare performance between the drug users in your organization and the non drug users. Well, if you take the time to figure who is using drugs, those employees probably are not going to continue their regular activities (the point of doing drug testing is to do something about it). Realistically, you may not be able to calculate a cost savings, but obviously, drug use is not consistent with a good working environment.

Some potential costs, monetary or otherwise, include:

Development and administration of a program. Writing a policy is a one time cost, but reviewing it regularly needs to occur. Further, other administrative costs are on-going. Someone has to maintain the policy and train employees. Someone has to address questions, handle problems and coordinate with other parties involved in testing.

Tangible cost of the test. Collection, analysis and MRO services are separate parts of the testing process, each may having its own fee. Expenses may average $50 per specimen.

Perception of employees. Many workers perceive drug testing to be invasive or unfair. However, quality drug testing programs that are implemented fairly are less likely to be perceived negatively. In many industries, drug testing is a way of life. You may be surprised to know that many workers expect to be tested.

Liability. A quality program is the best deterrent to liability issues. Nearly every aspect of the Federal DOT rules have been litigated and appealed; drug testing still takes place. Still, any employment practice can expose a business to liability. This must be weighed against liability from the public for negligent actions of employees who are under the influence.

Burden of record keeping. Records need to be retained for some period of time. DOT regulated programs have requirements. For unregulated testing, retaining records as long as other personnel information serves as a good rule of thumb. Under most circumstances, drug test results would not be considered part of an employee health record. Still, the results need to be confidential.

THE DRUG POLICY

Having a Policy

The importance of this document cannot be overstated. It may be required by one of the entities mentioned above or may just be part of your overall company policies. It also serves as guiding document when questions arise. If you are ever challenged about your drug testing, inevitably your policy will be a starting point. Besides having one, it is good practice to review it from time to time (e.g., at least once a year) so it can be updated. To me, the issue is not whether to have one, it is how much should it contain and what should be in it. Incidentally, a policy should be in place even if you do not perform drug testing. In this scenario, it would describe your company's position on drug use. This could serve to meet your obligations under the Drug Free Workplace Act.

One of the nice things of writing policy for your company is that you can decide what is in it. Even for areas of practice that are regulated, employers usually enjoy tremendous latitude in terms of content. With privilege comes responsibility. If you indicate that something is company policy, then do it. Perhaps more tragic than not having a policy is having one and then disregarding it. Therefore, it does take some thought and experience to draft one. There are a couple of approaches for this.

One solution is to take one already in existence. This is not as unscrupulous as it sounds. Many companies sell off-the-shelf products like this. A typical kit includes the policy, forms, usually a few flowcharts, and instructions. More and more are available on CD-Rom or other electronic formats. Hey, if it is on CD or the internet, it has got to be good. These usually run from $200-$400. You can also read through the DOT regulations to get an idea of what items to address and write your own. The text is fairly tedious and not very exciting. On the other hand, the regulations give a very good idea of the extent of thought process that went into it. Most of you are not that interested, which is fine. If you do write your own, I would advise some caution. I am not the type to give you all of these horror stories and scare tactics to get you to retain a high priced consultant. In fact, you can get into trouble no matter what you do. Writing your own policy forces you to think through potential problems *before* they happen rather than after. It probably does not hurt to have someone else review it, though. The advice can well be worth the money.

Another approach is to pay someone to write it. This may be a lawyer, doctor, or anyone who has done it. Just because a person is a lawyer, don't assume drug testing is their area of interest. Likewise, many doctors don't deal with drug testing issues. No one is a licensed drug testing policy writer. You just have to ask and hope you like what you hear. How do the "professionals" do it? The text itself can start as a template. People who have experience with drug testing know what areas can be problematic. Hopefully, your consultant will address these with you. Likewise, if you hire someone to review your policy, they should have a good sense of what makes a good document. It is a lot like my high school composition class. The teacher could not tell us "do this, this and this to get an A," but when she read through the papers she knew which ones were A papers and which were C+ papers. She also could tell what aspects of the content or style influenced her opinion. She could also give suggestions to make it more coherent or flow better. Policy is the same thing; you can get a feel for what is good and what is not. A consultant should have some understanding about your business organization and how you operate. This is true of any project for which you hire someone. Conversely, you should have some understanding of how your policy writer came up with the document.

When I work with employers, I make it collaborative. Always, I start with their current policy and their current practices, which are not always the same. The employer should have some understanding of what they want to accomplish and what can be achieved with a just a policy or a full program. I have to take into account the impact of drug use in their workforce, distribution of workforce, and the employer's ability (or willingness) to implement it. The company has to live with it and the policy is for them, not me. I try to clarify practices that are pretty standard and where things are truly dealer's choice. I also talk about where the company may be going a bit wayward in their intent. For example, unrealistic expectations are not uncommon. I cannot guarantee a perfect system and I cannot ensure that the employer will be drug free. Drug testing is a deterrent, not an insurance policy. Too often, an organization does not see the value of being educated and they just want the policy. The whole process just works better when management is actively involved in the process.

Contents of a Policy

There is, of course, different content from policy to policy and there is no one correct answer. The art of policy writing lies in the ability to capture pertinent information in as little space as possible. The level of detail definitely influences brevity. However, if the language is too generalized the employees will have difficulty understanding it, managers will have problems applying it and the employer won't be able to enforce it. If the language is too detailed, then even small variations in procedure will essentially put the employer out of compliance with their own policy! A detailed policy also requires the employer to address every possible scenario, which means that there is no ability to handle new situations that arise. In general, though, you want to address: scope, prohibited behaviors, procedure for testing, consequences for violating, and define responsibilities of management. Before addressing each of these, we need to look at more of the nuts and bolts of drug testing.

Scope

This lists which employees are covered by the policy. If certain groups are covered, then ensure that the policy provides an adequate description of who they are (job title, department, etc.). The scope section can mention the type of testing done (pre-employment, e.g.) as well as a reason for having the policy. Specific training about substance abuse is part of most drug testing programs. Training materials may be live presentations at orientation or distributing written information. Training methods should be discussed somewhere in the document.

Prohibited Behavior/Activity

This area discusses what you are regulating, which is generally phrased in terms of negatives or prohibitions. Employers need to ensure that the activity is something that they are able to detect and is a behavior that is under the employee's control. Simply being objective will prevent most problems. Most often you are prohibiting use of alcohol or illicit substances. Some employers emphasize or regulate the effects of drugs instead. For example, an employer might indicate that employees who make mistakes because of drugs may be terminated. The difficulty with this approach is that the employer must now link the event with drug use. If it is a pre-employment test, then you would have to prove the person's work capacity was limited. If it is a random test, you would have a similar burden of showing that the person had made some mistake or acted inappropriately. You now have three hurdles to clear before disciplining the employee: 1) Demonstrating that the person had an illegal substance in their body 2) Demonstrating that an accident or mistake had occurred 3) Demonstrating that the illegal substance was the reason for the accident. Compare this to an employer who prohibits the use of an illegal substance—this employer does not have the second or third hurdle to contend with.

Frequently, we use terms like "impairment" or "intoxication" to describe the effects of drugs. You will see these terms in books, in magazine articles, in company policies, or in regulatory text. Unfortunately, these terms are used by different entities to describe very different circumstances. Some entities even use them interchangeably, which is nothing less than confusing. Because the use of these terms is not universal, be sure that you define these terms, use them consistently, and use different terms for different concepts. This point is also discussed in the section on drug test results. Intoxication is often defined by legal authorities. For example, blood alcohol of .08% is legal intoxication in many states; its definition may also include other substances. The definition may exclude medication taken under the direction of a physician. Thus, if a person is using Vicodin® (a prescription pain medication) that his doctor gave him, he cannot be intoxicated based on that definition. Impairment can mean that a person is merely altered in some fashion (thought process or behavior) or it could mean someone is not at their normal level of performance. It may be independent of whether he or she is intoxicated or independent of whether he or she has used any specific substances. Impairment is often thought of as some observable behavior (such as a stumbling).

Realize that impairment can involve very minor changes that the naked eye cannot detect. A mere slowing in reflexes may not be detectable without formal, elaborate testing. The slowing of reflexes can be because someone used marijuana. In this case, the person would be considered intoxicated because he used an illegal substance. Note that you do not have to show what effect the marijuana is having. Marijuana is an illegal substance, the person used it and you found it in their system. This is sufficient to enforce most drug policies. A fairly common argument of drug users is that the marijuana, or whatever drug, found in their body was from use days ago. Further, the person may claim that it was not affecting them. As you can see, this rationale has no effect in what action is taken. Alternatively, a person could have altered performance, such as poor concentration, because of marital problems. This person could be considered impaired because his performance is altered, but would not be considered intoxicated.

In addition to prohibiting what type of activity is in violation of policy, a company must specify where the activity is prohibited. Of course, illicit drug use is prohibited "while a person is working." If we stop a moment, we can see that the definition may not be sufficient. For example, most organizations would not allow alcohol use on company property, including bathrooms, parking lots and cafeterias—regardless of whether the person is actively "working" or not. As you can see, your policy can fall victim to semantics. One of the best ways to avoid this is to define the terms you use. Regulating activity while traveling or while on-call at home should be addressed. Simple, common sense is usually adequate for these situations. You may have other policies from which you can borrow language.

Procedures for Testing

Here an employer describes issues such as who selects donors, how selection is done, mechanism to notify the employee for testing, and the obligation of the employee once notified. For purposes of your policy, the procedures do not have to be very detailed.

Consequences for Violating

Foremost in this section is to define what constitutes a violation. Usually, this is a positive test or refusing to take the test. The section on "Test Results" provides a full discussion on what makes a test positive. Consider it wise to structure the policy so that conditions not under the control of employee do not result in an adverse consequence. You will have a problem on your hands if an employee was not told to appear for a test and your policy requires you to suspend him for not showing. An employer may choose a zero tolerance approach where any positive test results in termination. Conversely, employers may have a "two strike" policy where an employee with a positive test is allowed an opportunity to undergo rehabilitation and a second positive test results in termination. The employee would be on leave (paid or nonpaid, depending on your benefits) during rehabilitation and would undergo accelerated testing once reinstated. This option requires a fair amount of expertise to coordinate the return to work issues. Many companies have adopted this approach because of the belief that drug or alcohol abuse is a medical problem. Doing nothing after a positive test or waiting for a second positive test probably has no role as a routine practice.

Handling of Results

The policy can indicate how results are stored and for how long. You should also address how results are released to the donor. In some circumstances, an organization may have a disclosure requirement to third parties because of a contractual obligation or a law covering certain professions. For example, you may have to report a positive test in a nurse to a nursing board. If the disclosure is due to a contractual obligation, you should ensure that the disclosure does not violate other laws, such as those that protect the employee's rights.

Management Responsibilities

An organization must determine who is responsible for administering the program, who will receive results, who will interact with third parties (e.g., the lab), and who can make decisions about problems that develop. Frequently, this individual will be someone who handles human resource issues. Larger organizations may have several people. Regardless, this person should be identified in the document, usually by title. Identifying one person rather than several will minimize ambiguity. If every manager had to train and select employees as well as handle drug test results, the organization will have a difficult time ensuring consistency.

Other Party Responsibilities

Because most, if not all, organizations will use other providers of services, the policy should mention their role. Companies usually do not collect urine and companies do not do their own testing. Other parties do this. Discussing the role of third parties demonstrates program integrity and can help provide assurance to skeptics. For example, stating that testing will be conducted by an accredited lab tells people about the high standards of your program. Likewise, results will be reviewed by a "physician who is a certified medical review officer" (discussed later). Many of these points are taken for granted, but they can serve as a selling point.

Maintaining standards like these are truly optional in many instances and your program probably is not deficient without these practices. However, they do emphasize the quality of your program. More and more often, though, they are becoming minimum standards. Be sure that all parties know what is expected of them. It makes no sense to say that the collection site will have the final review of the test result when, in fact, it does not.

Implementation and Education

An organization has to notify its employees of a policy or procedure that they are expected to follow. Typical education includes providing information about your policy as well as who is responsible for administering it, resources for treatment (if any), signs and symptoms of drug/alcohol use, and how to report suspicious behavior. Some of these components are required by the groups that regulate testing and some points are discretional. In cases where it is optional, an employer is not necessarily negligent for not showing a 30 minute video on the symptoms of glue sniffing. Yet, these aspects of training are found in many programs and there is little incremental burden in providing fairly comprehensive training. As an individual has more responsibility for administering the program, the amount of training should also increase. An employee who just needs to not use drugs and show up for testing when their supervisor tells them may not need much training beyond that. On the other hand, the supervisor who can send people for "for cause" testing needs more education such as how to identify someone properly. In essence, you should plan to have employee training and supervisor training. There is no reason that you could not incorporate the training into an employee meeting or combine it with other training. You should document all training.

Below is a summary of what to include in a substance abuse policy:

- Scope
- Prohibited behavior
- Testing procedures
- Consequences for violating
- Handling results
- Responsibility of management and third parties
- Implementation and education

DIFFERENT TIMES TO TEST SOMEONE

Selecting employees to be tested has to be done fairly. Nonetheless, the employer can still choose at what points a person is tested and, to a lesser extent, can decide which groups of employees can be tested. Commonly accepted types of testing are: Pre-employment, random, for cause, and post-accident.

Pre-employment testing—Testing that occurs in a job candidate/ new employee before he/she commences employment.

Random testing—Testing where selection occurs without a person being able to predict it.

Post Accident—Selection for testing is triggered by an event, in this case following accidents.

For cause—There is some behavior in an employee that warrants testing.

Now that you are familiar with some times when drug testing can occur, you will need to make some decisions about whether to do just one type of testing or to conduct all four types. This is influenced by cost, practicality and perception of problem. Let's look at each of these again, but in more detail.

Pre-Employment Testing

If you are going to have any sort of drug test, it makes sense that you should at least have pre-employment. So I will assume that you are doing this. Although the Americans with Disabilities Act (ADA) prohibits medical inquiries of applicants, drug testing for illegal substances is permitted at the pre-employment stage. From a practical standpoint, much pre-employment testing is done at the post-offer stage. I spoke earlier about the art of policy writing. Here is an example of my stylistic preferences. Rather than just stating in your policy that you will conduct pre-employment drug testing, spell it out. Define it somewhere in your policy so that there is no misunderstanding as to when pre-employment is. Also indicate who is tested pre-employment. Although most companies will test everybody across the board, they actually do not have to. It is permissible to test certain employees, as long they fit into a group that the employer has defined. For example, if you have a pizza shop, you could test everyone who will be a delivery driver. The trick is, you have to know who will be delivering pizzas. It seems straightforward, but envision where employees are cross-trained so that a person may take an order, cook the pizza, and possibly deliver it. You are back to pretty much testing everyone. Even if "delivery driver" is actually a separate title from "pizza cooker" you can run into problems. If the driver calls in sick and the manager would have to deliver pizzas, then you need to be sure to have tested the manager. What if a person who was a "pizza cooker" transfers into the "delivery driver" position? You need to address this. A policy cannot cover all possible situations, but a little forethought can address most scenarios.

The other bear trap is that selection can be discrimination, however so subtle. Let's say you have a cleaning business and you want to test only housekeepers. You do this because these housekeepers come in direct contact the public and even go into their houses. This is plausible, even to me. However, what are the demographics of housekeepers? Are they more likely to be a minority, women, or some other distinguishing group? It could be construed that your standard is a sham to just test women. Personally, I think testing housekeepers is a reasonable standard. Truthfully, you may never have a problem with it. But, there are people out there who have a lot of free time on their hands to think of reasons why you are discriminating. As you can see, I recommend testing everyone. I think it is more trouble than it is worth to test only subgroups. Nonetheless, in certain instances it may be appropriate. If you do test certain groups, ensure that you have a rational, business purpose underlying your choice.

It is as important to mention some inappropriate criteria for determining who gets tested. You cannot make a determination on a case by case basis. Let's say you open a restaurant and you hire 10 people for waiters/waitresses. You could not interview people and decide that those who gave marginal answers (but nonetheless hired) would get tested. This is just too subjective. Even some predefined criteria can cause more headaches than it is worth. Testing applicants who did not finish high school could be one instance. A high school diploma is a objective, verifiable endpoint. Yet, it lacks a rationale basis. You could try to link high school drop out rates to drug use, but this is a fairly tangential thought process to justify not doing testing across the board. Clearly, your legal counsel may feel otherwise. From the perspective of how things are just done, it is an all or none phenomenon when dealing with subsets of people.

Having said all this, testing only some groups of employees does happen in the real world. The U.S. Department of transportation does not require testing of everyone who works for a trucking company. It is mandated only for those are required to have a commercial driver's license. The FAA includes airline mechanics in its scope. The distinguishing factor is that these employees fill safety sensitive positions (a valid business purpose). In these circumstances, testing only some employees works fairly well. The DOT (and their agencies) took the time to define terms and to address potential problems. It also took years to draft the final rule.

Random Testing

Many of the concepts discussed in the pre-employment section also apply to random testing. It is not unusual to find companies that do pre-employment testing, but not random. This does not indicate a weak program. Random testing is harder to implement and manage than is pre-employment testing. Obviously, the principle behind random testing is that unscheduled testing is more likely to deter drug use. There is rationale, likewise, that someone could stay clean long enough to test negative at the start of employment, hence beating the dragon. This is probably not the entire story as there are other dynamics in place. Even with open policies about drug testing (i.e., telling a person that he/she will be tested on Tuesday when they come in to fill out an application), people still test positive. I have commented to many people that drug testing is in part an IQ test. You tell someone that they will be tested, how hard can it be? In actual fact, some people do not understand how drug testing works, what will trigger a positive test, and what are the consequences of a positive test. Without getting into a deep debate about what makes a drug user different from non-drug users, I think most authorities would agree that the behavioral aspects of the user are important when trying to understand drug use and abuse. Part of this behavior can include features of denial and invincibility. Drug users and abusers may not see getting caught as a possibility. The invincibility trait is reinforced when a person continues to use and does not experience what they perceive as a consequence. Here, it means they have not tested positive. Let's just jump to the other end of the spectrum—some people don't care if they get caught. Some people assume that even if the test is positive it will have no effect unless use is at work.

This can explain in part why some companies do only pre-employment. With random testing, it takes more energy and money to find drug users. Even if it is more labor intensive to administer, it is worth considering. First, the extra time and money does not automatically make random testing prohibitive. Random testing is consistent with a corporate philosophy of not tolerating drug use. It also shows diligence of an employer to deter drug use; words and policy have only a limited effect.

OK, you are sold on random testing. We can look at some of the more technical aspects, starting with random. When we apply randomness to drug testing, we do mean lacking predictability. You do not have to hire statisticians or draw Gaussian curves. You can literally pull names out of a hat, use a random number generator, or use a list of names on a spreadsheet. As long as a person cannot predict who will get picked and there is not human bias, it is probably acceptable. If you pull names out of a hat, then mix up the hat before selecting and make sure the bits of paper are the same size. If you have lists of names, don't have someone look at the list to select people. That introduces bias into the selection process. Conversely, picking the first person of the shift who uses the coffee machine on the morning following a new moon is very objective, but predictable. OK, not obviously so. You get the point.

Reselection is also important. If employee 31 is selected for a drug test today, the next time you drug test be sure that employee 31 has as good a chance as anyone else of being selected. Be sure to randomize the selection of testing dates and times. Choosing people every Monday is not very random.

How often you do random testing will vary depending on how many random tests you plan to do. Usually, this is expressed as a minimum percentage of the workforce (or size of random pool if you test only certain groups). If everyone can potentially be randomly tested and there are 50 workers, you might randomly test at least 20% a year (10 people for the liberal arts readers). For example, the DOT agencies publish the minimum percentages each year in the *Federal Register*. The percentage varies according to the previous year's positive rates and usually is between 10% and 25%. Bear in mind that in order to test 10 people, you may actually have to select 15 or 20 since some people take vacation or are not at work. Some companies will select additional names, while others just over select to be sure they hit their minimum testing target. I do not have a particular preference, just be consistent.

Your policy should indicate that you do random testing (assuming you do random test) and give some information as to how. Listing every painful detail of the process is not necessary in your document. Saying something like, "At different intervals, the Director of Human Resources will select the names of employees for random drug testing. Selection is done using software with randomization features . . ." You probably should have a fairly detailed list of instructions regarding the exact process, but you may wish to have this only as part of a manual for the employee who does the selection. This is not to hide the document or prevent employees from "discovering" your system. It is just a practical matter which prevents cluttering of your corporate policies. Consider the difficulty in revising your entire drug policy because of a few minor changes in methods. You would have to redistribute your policy to all of your workforce rather than just update an instruction sheet. The trend in testing is to outsource the random selection process. This removes human bias from the process.

Also mention in your policy what happens when employees do not show up for testing. Their reason for failing to appear may be valid or invalid. A person who is on vacation when called or a person who says "I refuse to get tested" are the easiest situations to handle. Everything else in between is much tougher. Some people will not be able to get away for testing. If there is a chemical leak in your warehouse, then the person who is your paramedic may not be able to leave. Do not try to list every possible circumstance that can arise. Language like "Not presenting for testing is acceptable if their absence from the worksite is likely to compromise the safety of others or adversely affect core operations . . ."

will convey the idea and give some leeway. Place a time limit on how long an employee is allowed to take to go to the test site (e.g., 2 hours).

You should be explicit about who decides that it is acceptable for someone not to get tested upon being selected. The employee should not make this determination for himself. Even an immediate supervisor may not be sufficient. The issue of favoritism can arise. If your company has four managers with three employees each and you have delegated the power to excuse to the managers, an employee can claim he is being picked on because his work is just as critical and that his co worker did not have to get tested when called. The structure of your business can make the manager the only practical choice, though. For example, you own 5 dry cleaning shops, each with a manager. The store manager is obviously the best person to decide what is too disruptive to business. One way to reduce the favoritism risk, real or perceived, is to require the manager to talk to someone higher up. Simple statement : " . . . where the manager determines the employee's temporary absence . . . the manager will discuss the situation with the Director of Human Resources . . ." Document the nature of events.

The above considerations point to some of the reasons some companies do not have random testing in their program. Logistically, it is much tougher to implement than pre-employment.

Post Accident

I will mention post-accident testing only briefly. The biggest chore is to establish what constitutes an accident. Filling out an incident report does not always imply an accident occurred; it could represent a situation. Most organizations encourage reporting near miss situations and would not want to punish someone for speaking up. On the other hand, at some point it becomes an accident? Now someone needs to determine if it constitutes an accident. This will introduce some human bias to the process. Interestingly, OSHA had indicated, in their preamble to the now repealed ergonomic standard, that post-accident drug testing can serve as a disincentive for employees to report unsafe conditions; discouraging this reporting can lead to an OSHA citation. Accidents also inherently assign blame. An employee who slips on a wet floor clearly had an accident. Most companies that test post accident would test the employee who slipped. If she did not know the floor was wet because someone else did not use a sign, then you will be testing the wrong employee. Some accidents occur due to equipment malfunction. You end up punishing someone because they are convenient to identify, but there is not really a better way to handle this. In any case, most post-accident criteria I see involve some estimated cost in dollars (e.g., estimated damage over $300). Criteria can be experiencing a specific number of accidents in a 3 or 6 month period. As general advice, if you utilize post-accident testing identify fairly discrete situations.

For Cause

For cause testing should be part of most drug testing programs. This is true even if an organization decides not to do pre-employment or random testing. It actually is a different animal from other types of drug testing. Assessing observed behavior is the underlying motive in for cause testing, whereas deterrence underlies pre-employment and random testing. Whereas, pre-employment and random serve to deter drug use, for cause testing is more diagnostic. Basically, someone suspects that use may contribute to a performance problem. Sometimes the performance issue is abrupt. Staggered walking, shaking, falling asleep at a workstation would fall into this category. The performance issue can actually be a series of events over time. Erratic work output, complaints from customers, missed deadlines can be a symptom of drug use, but really require a pattern of behavior rather than a single incident to suggest the problem is other than a bad hair day.

It is important to identify what behaviors can trigger testing. I like checklists. This ensures that each potential donor receives a similar assessment. Treating everyone the same is key in human resources. Leaving a space for comments is a good idea. Documenting as much detail as possible will serve in the employer's interest. Try to document behavior and not conclusions. When you say a person is not able to stand, you remain objective. When you say, "employee appears drunk," it is more presumptive. List witnesses, times, and places.

Part of your protocol should be identifying who bears the responsibility for ordering a for cause test. Frequently, more than one person may have to verify the behavior. Realizing that much behavior may be noted by customers or co-workers, create a mechanism to funnel those complaints to someone in a management position.

Most behavior suggestive of drug or alcohol use is nonspecific. Shaking and confusion can result from severe infections. Poor performance can result from family troubles or other stressors. Thus, for cause testing is frequently one aspect of a fitness for duty evaluation. Whether a company has an employee assistance program (EAP) will influence the mechanism of steps. The usual process involves a manager (employee relations, if a separate function) confronting the employee about performance. The employee is sent for either a drug test, an evaluation by a physician, or both. The rationale for sending the employee for a medical exam is to rule out a life threatening cause. Simply put, it would be really devastating to smell what you think is alcohol on someone's breath, send him home and have him die because it was actually his presentation for new onset diabetes. Sending the employee for a medical evaluation also provides an objective, outside, professional opinion. Some employers leave the decision of whether a drug test is necessary to the examiner; others test regardless of the outcome of the evaluation. Either approach is acceptable.

As an employment practice, mandatory medical exams warrant a word of caution since they can be construed as punitive. After all, you are requiring a person to submit to something that can have a negative effect on them. Employers must maintain a pretty high threshold before subjecting someone for a required evaluation by a physician or an EAP counselor. This is one area where mere concern of a person's well being can get you into trouble. The decision to initiate a visit must be based on a legitimate business necessity. For a single episode, the behavior should be near extreme and for a pattern of behavior, it should be well documented and recurrent. On the other hand, there is nothing that prevents you from counseling a person about their performance. However, there should be some distance between saying a person's work performance is not good and saying the performance is not good AND that it may be due to a substance abuse problem. Required evaluations require balancing the rights of employees against the interests of an organization.

Now that you have diligently concluded that someone gets a for cause test, what happens after testing? The answer probably relates more to how your organization handles lost time than how it handles drug testing. One thing is clear—if a person is staggering or sleeping at their desk, he or she should not be at work regardless of the cause. The issue is whether there is a punitive action or not. It may be three days before the drug test is back. You may not want to suspend without pay someone who had stroke at work, but you thought they were on marijuana.

A couple of common alternatives include either suspending all such people with pay or to treat the absence as a sick day. In a union environment, the former is fairly common. Additionally, suspension of employees, particularly exempt (salaried) employees, can raise Wage and Hour issues. Quite honestly, this will not come up much so you are spending a lot of time to figure out how you can save $400 a year. Whomever structures your benefits and lost time procedures will be in the best position to address this. More importantly, indicate to employees what will happen.

Below is a summary of when to do drug testing:

- Pre-employment testing
- Random testing
- Post-accident testing
- For Cause

OTHER PARTIES IN DRUG TESTING

Once you have decided to have drug testing, there are three other parties who are likely to participate. 1) A collection site 2) A medical review officer 3) A laboratory

Collection Site

Unless you have in-house medical facilities, you probably won't be performing the actual collection of urine specimens from candidates/employees. Urine specimens used in employment drug testing are not like a urine sample you give the doctor at a physical. It is not as simple as having the payroll clerk distribute containers and subsequently pick them up an hour later. Urine, for employment purposes, is more like "evidence" in that it is collected under a chain of custody. A collector does not have to be a doctor or nurse, but it is doubtful that another employee will do it. It is just too weird. Some people are in the business of doing nothing but collecting urine specimens. Most clinics that cater to worker's compensation or occupational medicine will offer urine collection services. $25 is an approximate charge for just the collection. Proper collection is extremely important to the drug testing process. Improper collection can result in a test being cancelled or in a test result that cannot be defended. Urinating into a cup has become quite a science. Basic steps include confirming the identity of the donor, deterring adulteration of specimen, and packaging/shipping the container to the lab. With each of these steps, there are (should be) procedures for when things don't go right.

Verifying ID is pretty straightforward. As an employer, you can pick forms of ID which are acceptable, usually an official picture ID or company badge. For those who amazingly have no photo ID, a company official can vouch for their identity.

The collector will either give the donor a container or allow him to select one. Allowing someone to select the cup rather than giving them one is one of those subtleties of urine collection that you would swear was contrived by someone with too much time on their hands. Someone who is given a container can claim they were "set-up" or given one that was spiked with drugs. Likewise, the container should be sealed. The donor goes into the bathroom and fills the cup. Privacy should be afforded. Except rare, specific circumstances, people are not observed while giving a specimen. It may not necessarily be a legal reason as much as it is a social reason. When I was a medical student, I used to watch people giving specimens for employment drug testing. It was not quite how my mother envisioned her son, the doctor, to be spending his days. Then drug testing was a fairly new game and witnessed specimens were more common. Since then, practices have evolved. The primary reason to witness a specimen was to prevent someone from introducing a fake specimen. Other mechanisms are in place now to deter this.

Although interesting, listing all of the finer points of how proper collection procedures minimize altering a specimen is too cumbersome. I will mention some quick points. Usually the toilet room will not have a sink in it. If there is a sink, the water should be turned off. Colored dye is placed into the bowl and the donor is instructed not to flush until after the specimen is sealed. The collector will measure the temperature range of the specimen. These steps help to deter adulteration. Really, pretty dry stuff, but it is fairly standard in the business. Below lists some of the common problems that can arise in collecting a specimen. Only a brief description of the solution is provided. Suffice it to say that standard practices may be rather detailed. Although your personnel may not be urine collectors, knowing about these issues will help you identify a good collection site.

No show or refusal to give specimen	This is handled as if the person has a positive test. Stating this in a policy is a good idea.
No ID	A company representative can vouch for someone's identity
Cannot give specimen	Usually the person is given water and told to wait until they can produce a specimen. The specifics of this are not important here

Refusal to sign a chain of custody; Ignores instructions (e.g., does not wash hands); General conduct issues	I lumped these together since they are handled similarly. The specimen is submitted and tested, but a comment is made, indicating the behavior, on the chain of custody

Key to the collection process is the "chain of custody" (COC) form. This creates the paper trail for documenting a good procedure. In essence, the COC links a specific specimen to a specific person. A drug test report will have some identifier on it, but frequently not a name (again, to eliminate bias). Without a COC, a donor could claim the laboratory tested a different bottle or that the collector switched bottles. The COC prevents this. The COC has several copies since the donor, collector, and the other players get a copy. The COC starts at collection, follows the specimen to the lab, continues to the MRO at the time of verification, and is ultimately filed. The donor signs the form to indicate that the specimen is his. A donor also initials a seal that is placed over the container to seal it. The collector, as well as any other person who handles the specimen, signs the form as well. Because the container is sealed within a shipping package, the kind people who ship the specimen do not sign the form. There are check boxes to indicate ID was verified and that the specimen was within temperature range. An improperly completed COC can invalidate a test result!

Tips to Evaluate Collection Site:

- What is the overall appearance of the facility?
- How do they train collectors?
- Do they have standardized forms?
- Are collection procedures written?
- How do they handle employees without an ID or who cannot produce a specimen?
- How well do they communicate with their clients?

Laboratory

The laboratory, of course, tests the specimen. First, they ensure that the container is intact and that the chain of custody form has accompanied the specimen. Testing is very automated and is very accurate. The test performed is actually a screening test. If it is negative, then the lab issues a test result stating it is "negative." A typical process tests for 5-15 drug groups and the specimen is screened for all. If there is something detected (i.e., positive), the specimen is retested for that drug using a different, much more specific test. It is actually quicker, cheaper, and more reliable to conduct testing like this rather than just using one step testing. The screening test is quick. However, it is likely to "flag" some samples that don't actually have drugs in them. A screening test could actually detect some things other than what it intends to. It is not a bad method, it is just that the test was not designed to test only for one specific substance or some substances can interfere with it. Only after being confirmed with the second test will the result be reported as positive. Laboratories frequently allow the client to have only the screening test performed. These positive results rarely are sufficient for employment purposes and I discourage them.

The lab does some quick tests to see if the specimen is adulterated. Specific gravity and pH are the most common. Urine has a certain range of normal density and pH, results outside these bounds may very well indicate that the container does not contain just urine. The lab may also comment on the smell, color or gross appearance (I have not found one to comment on taste) of the urine. Any remarks about unusual characteristics should be followed up with an objective test. Saying "scientifically validated" sounds so much more impressive. Results are sent to whomever you designate and should be your MRO (discussed later).

Although most medical laboratories can perform tests for drugs, not all utilize strict chain of custody procedures. This special handling is essential in employment drug testing. Still, no one will have a problem finding a good lab. DOT mandated specimens must be tested in an DHHS approved laboratory; there are about 70 in the country. The approved labs will also test non Federal specimens utilizing the same procedures. The DHHS rules for labs are very stringent and minimize the mishandling of specimens and bias. Further, the labs are required to undergo inspection and reaccreditation. Labs must have quality assurance procedures and have competent personnel. As you can see, there is a lot of quality assurance built into the certified lab. You can use other laboratories for non-DOT specimens. Many non certified labs are good;

it is just harder to figure which ones are the good ones. Finding a local lab is not essential because shipping is easy to do. The bigger labs accept specimens from all over the country, but may actually test specimens at only one or two locations. Processing time is not usually an issue and 2-3 day turnaround times are the norm; competition has brought about incredible efficiency in the system.

Beyond the basics of selecting a lab, some minor criteria can be helpful. I will actually review laboratory reports to see if the layout is clear. Reviewing standard language on the report is helpful. Reports will frequently print that they are HHS certified on the report and also indicate GC/MS (gas chromatography or mass spectrometry) confirmation is done automatically for positive screens. These statements add a little credibility to the testing.

With drug test adulteration remaining a concern, I like to know what capabilities a lab has for testing and how it prints those results. Remember, as an MRO, I can address adulteration results that used a scientifically valid method. I can't do anything with vague laboratory language. The above issues do not occur frequently and it may not be worth the time to address a problem that may never arise. However, when they do occur, they are very labor intensive. The bottom line is that it is worthwhile to have a good lab.

Medical Review Officer (MRO)

The medical review officer determines if the final result is negative or positive for a urine drug test. OK, the lab sends out a sheet of paper that says "negative" or "positive;" why would you pay someone to "interpret" this? It is entirely possible to have a result come from the lab as "positive," but for the final answer to be "negative." First, the MRO ensures that the chain of custody was not violated. An incomplete chain of custody can invalidate a test result. The bigger reason for having an MRO is that the role of a lab is different from the role of the drug test itself. The lab is commenting on whether or not they *detected*, using a scientific method, the substance. Employment drug testing is designed to detect *illicit* substances. Thus, the MRO must incorporate medical information and seek whether there is a valid, medical reason for why the substance is present. As an MRO, I do this by understanding the testing process, the nature of the drugs tested for, and what constitutes valid use. Standards for an MRO would include actually speaking to the donor (some exceptions exist) before rendering a positive test decision. An MRO can also resolve some problems that arise during testing and can serve as a resource for questions.

The Department of Transportation and some states require the use of an MRO. Further, these agencies set criteria for who can act as an MRO. An MRO is a physician who has knowledge of substance abuse issues and an understanding of pharmacology. There are organizations that provide formalized training and certification to physicians. More and more states are requiring that an MRO be certified or at least receive formal training. Although the majority of physicians have some experience in diagnosing and treating substance abusers, most do not have a solid background in employment drug testing. Standard practices in urinary drug test programs are not part of the standard curriculum in medical schools. To be an MRO, a physician must have an understanding of the drug testing process and not just the effect of drugs on a person.

TEST RESULTS

Negative Result

This deserves special attention because misconceptions are somewhat commonplace. When the laboratory reports a negative result, the test is negative. Fairly easy. A negative specimen has a few different meanings. It does mean that the substances for which the tests are designed to detect were not detected. It does not mean that person has not used any illicit substance. You could not design a testing panel that could detect *every* possible impairing substances. A negative result could mean that a person did have an illicit substance in his/her body, but its concentration was below the level of detection. A negative test does not mean that a person was not impaired.

Positive Result

Positive tests can be a little more difficult to understand. First, the language is ambiguous. Positive can refer to the laboratory result or to the MRO final determination, which can be different. Once the laboratory determines that a result is positive, it is up to the MRO to decide if the final result will be positive or negative (there is a "cancelled specimen" option, but this is uncommon and usually due to procedural errors). An MRO positive result indicates that the laboratory detected a substance and the MRO concluded that there was no legitimate medical explanation for it. A typical MRO report to the employer will give the date of the test and indicate which substance for which it was positive. Some MROs will indicate the drug level, but this is not very meaningful. In fact, many labs do not print the concentration of the drug. The lab report just says "positive." Since there is a cut-off level, any drug detected was at least that level.

Perhaps a bigger area of confusion is understanding some things that a positive test does not tell us. A positive test does not indicate when a person used the substance. Drugs metabolize at different rates in different people. All you can determine is that the substance detected was present in the donor's body at the time of collection. Based on metabolism, a typical substance could have been present for up to a few days after use. The medical literature debates for how long a substance can be detected, but up to 3 days or 5 days is commonly accepted. A positive result does not tell us the effect of a drug on a particular person.

A drug test does not tell you how a person was behaving or performing at the time of collection. People tend to confuse impairment with use. Impairment relates more to how a person is behaving or how the person is affected. Drug tests tell us which drugs are present, not how impaired a person is. Fortunately, your company policy states that the use of illicit substances is prohibited. A drug test performed in a scientific manner proves that use occurred so you do not even need to address impairment. From my standpoint, the mere use of illegal drugs is impairing. This is why quantitative levels are superfluous. If an airline pilot were to have cocaine in his system, he would not be allowed to fly. No one would check to see to what extent it was affecting his ability to fly; the pilot just would not be permitted to sit in the cockpit. A cocaine level of 1000 is not twice as bad, twice as impairing or twice as positive as a level of 500—it is positive. Further, the outcome is not contingent upon the level in that you cannot fire a person twice.

Explanations For Laboratory Positives

Another point of caution regards lab positive specimens that the MRO reports as negative, so-called downgrades. Recall this occurs when there is a legitimate medical explanation for the presence of the detected drug. Once the laboratory has detected a substance and issues a positive report, there are two ways to look at the verification process. One is to put the burden upon the employee to provide information to support that the drug use is medically legitimate and the other is to put the burden upon the MRO to show that the drug use is *not* from legitimate use. In practice, it is a little bit of both based upon which drug was detected and the MRO. PCP has no legitimate uses (in people); the burden is fully on the employee to show otherwise. Benzodiazepines (such as Valium®) have lots of legitimate uses; the MRO has some burden. Basically, the person (donor) is given the opportunity to provide an explanation.

While it may seem like an MRO is giving information to the donor that allows the donor to answer "correctly", the donor still has to provide documentation. A sense of fairness comes into play as well. The MRO has knowledge of the pharmacology and medical uses of various drugs whereas a donor may not. Envision what would happen if a specimen contained opiates and the donor was given pain medication during a dental procedure. If the MRO does not ask, the donor may not think to mention it. This would turn drug testing into a quiz of the donor's fund of knowledge in pharmaceuticals. Overall, the burden is on the donor. The MRO just gives the donor an opportunity to provide documentation. The MRO should review the documentation. What the MRO accepts is a matter of professional judgment. Prescriptions are written by a practitioner and filled by a pharmacy; this can be verified. Medication given during a procedure can be verified. A person who went to an emergency room, received something there, but cannot recall which hospital, has not really provided documentation.

In practice, many organizations do not like the idea that a "positive" test can be reported as "negative." Thus, some organizations like to receive the results directly. Their stance is that anyone who takes codeine or who takes benzodiazepines is not fit to work. This is a very difficult position to justify. Such blanketing prohibitions can end up punishing unintended parties. Excluding groups of people based on this type of medical criteria is at odds with the Americans with Disabilities Act (ADA). Another approach adopted by organization to deal with this problem of downgrades is to put additional burdens on the employee. Companies have done everything including mandating that the drug levels be below a certain amount, requiring additional performance testing or requiring letters from their physician. Overall, these are not mainstream, accepted industry practices and any group wishing to implement these solutions should confer with their legal advisors. Most MROs simply do not report that a specimen was downgraded, rather the MRO merely reports "positive" or "negative." From a company's perspective, it should not matter. So, it is not worth asking.

Below I provide some examples of explanations that a donor may give for a positive result. While each situation requires an individual assessment of the available information, I provide my general rationale for each. This is not intended to provide specific guidance to anyone for interpreting drug test results. Each instance needs to be reviewed separately.

"I was at a concert/club/party and other people were using [marijuana]"	Under typical second hand exposure conditions, concentrations in the donor's system would be below the testing cutoff. Thus, levels above the cutoff represent use
"I used my wife's/husband's medication last night because…"	Medication is prescribed to an individual, not a household. Thus, using medication prescribed to another is illicit use. The DOT does not recognize spousal use as a legitimate medical explanation. This occurs with some regularity. I encourage companies to address this in their policy.
"Can I retest?"	No rationale for retesting if the test was performed by a scientifically valid method. Hence, the importance of having solid collection and testing procedures.
"I bought the medication over-the-counter in Canada/Mexico and brought it back with me."	In the U.S., these are prescription medications. Unless, the person declared them to customs upon entry, it is not legitimate. I encourage organizations to include this explicitly in their policy.
"I was not impaired at the time [of collection]."	Irrelevant. It is the use of illicit substances that is prohibited; not its effect. Further, one argument is that the use of illicit substances is, by definition, impairing.
"I have had other negative drug tests recently"	It does not mean anything. Separate tests are interpreted independently.

One other common explanation provided by donors is that something "else" caused the test to be positive. For example, someone may claim that over the counter decongestants made the test positive for amphetamines or that they received lidocaine during a dental procedure that must have caused the test to be positive for cocaine. These assertions are largely without merit, but need to be reviewed based on the individual facts and circumstances of each. An MRO should be able to make a determination without much of a problem.

The outcome of a drug test decision can have a significant impact on a person's life—specifically, they may lose a job. All the issues of discrimination, wrongful termination and defamation of character apply to drug testing. If I were telling a person that you won't hire them because of a drug test result (and in essence, saying that they used drugs), I would want the process to be flawless. These procedures bring you a little closer to perfection. Managers become frustrated when employees appear to "beat the system." A positive result that isn't credible is not worth having.

Adulterated Tests

Under limited circumstances, a few other results can occur with a drug test. The MRO may report the test as cancelled. In this case, usually an administrative error has occurred and this creates doubt regarding the reliability of the test. Cancelled tests are not very common. If you see more than one, it may represent a problem with the collection site.

The laboratory may report that the specimen shows signs of adulteration. This is more difficult for an MRO to handle. The report may comment on an usual odor or may actual have tested for adulterating substances. Suspecting adulteration lacks enough information to say that the specimen is adulterated. It is enough to perform further testing on the specimen. A test (or group of tests) that demonstrates adulteration is obviously sufficient. Your policy should state that adulterating a test is a refusal to take a test. Refusing to take a test is treated like a positive. By the way, suspicion by the collector, rather than the laboratory, would not justify special testing.

Adulteration has been occurring as long as drug testing has been taking place. It represents a developing area in the science of drug testing, though, because of the advances in testing itself. If you search the internet or read through enough magazines, you will see businesses that sell drug adulteration kits. Adulteration does not cause an otherwise negative test to become positive, only positive tests become negative. Undoubtedly, people do fool the drug test enough that it cannot be called positive. Overall, however people who run drug testing programs are smarter than people who use the drugs and adulterate the specimen.

Using the Test Result and Personnel Actions

Now that you have gone through all of these previous steps to ensure you have a solid drug testing program, you now have to do something with results. Below are a few possible alternatives.

If you have a positive test result, one option is to terminate a person. By positive I am referring to a final, confirmed positive. It is entirely acceptable to fire someone who tests positive. Like any other employer policy, a violation of it could result in termination. Recall that your policy is prohibiting (illicit) drug use. So, you are firing someone for violating that policy. You do not have to show what type of affect the drug is having on the person; this can be quite difficult if not impossible in many situations. This demonstrates the importance of prohibiting the use of drugs, rather that prohibiting a person from having a certain impairment/affect from a drug. Certain states may have laws addressing this or a collective bargaining agreement have contain other provisions. You should ensure that any of your employment policies are consistent with these regulations or agreements.

A different option is to permit a person to undergo rehabilitation and re-enter the workplace clean and drug free. Of course, the person is taken off work until rehabilitated. This option is fairly labor intensive. However, it recognizes that drug abuse is a medical condition, like heart disease or diabetes. This approach creates several new issues as well, such as who pays for the treatment and whether the person is put on paid leave while in treatment. Probably the easiest solutions are to handle this kind of leave the same as any other medical leave. Thus, a person could use remaining sick days with pay and any remaining time as unpaid leave. It makes sense to have the employee maintain financial responsibility for their treatment. So, if you offer health insurance, then it would have some coverage for drug rehabilitation.

Record Keeping

All results should be kept in confidential files. Then again, so should all personnel records and medical records. Only specified individuals should have access. Positive results and negative results should be retained. Consulting state labor laws is a good place to start. Some organizations retain results for the length of employment, others keep results for a specified length of time (e.g., one year for negatives). Besides the individual results, aggregate data should also be kept. This includes lists of persons in the random pool, the number of persons selected and the number of persons actually tested. Unless there is law elsewhere, many organizations keep the test result for the same length of time as other employment records.

WHICH DRUGS SHOULD I TEST FOR?

Again, for those who have Department of Transportation mandated programs, the Government has removed this decision for us. It must be the "NIDA-5"—marijuana, cocaine, PCP, opiates, and amphetamines. Most laboratories offer a few standard panels in addition to the NIDA-5. Panels which test for seven, nine or ten drugs are fairly common. These will test for benzodiazepines, Darvocet® and other commonly used drugs. There are even customized panels, such as those which cater to the medical profession by testing for drugs like Vicodin® or Fentanyl®. Unless you are in a business or geographic area where a specific drug is in especially high use, standard panels should be sufficient. Nine drug panels usually are not much more expensive than a five drug panels, so many employers get the biggest panel for the lowest price. The only downside is that you will find more legally used drugs. Remember, a legally used drug will result in a negative drug test. Each test that comes back from the lab with a detected substance has to be addressed on an individual basis. So, there is more time needed to administer your testing program. Time is money. Inevitably, some employers take inappropriate actions, e.g. termination or suspension, based on the laboratory result only. There is some merit in not looking too hard. If you test for marijuana and cocaine, you will find most of what is being used.

ALCOHOL TESTING

How It Differs From Other Drug Testing

Alcohol deserves some special comments because it is a legal substance. As an employer, it is difficult to regulate a person's use of alcohol while the employee is not at work. This is obviously different from illegal substances. It is permissible to fire a person based on finding marijuana in their system. Their actual use may have been two days ago, but it does not matter. The termination occurs because they used marijuana, an illegal substance, not because of when they used it. To be meaningful, alcohol test results need to reflect recent use. Urine alcohol is worthless in employment drug testing programs. The only thing it means is that the person had some alcohol in the last couple of days. In fact, I request that labs not print the urine alcohol result because I don't know what to do with it. Realize that urine alcohol is reliable, but it just does not provide useful information. It would be difficult to justify taking a personnel action because someone drank wine over the weekend. This would be a pretty common explanation for positive urine alcohols.

In addition to being a legal substance, alcohol testing differs from illegal substance testing for a couple other reasons as well. Most obvious is that the test is usually a breath test rather than urine. Next, the results are available immediately which means there is no necessary involvement of an MRO. However, some organizations choose to have a health care professional review the results.

Next, many organizations have different consequences based on the different cutoff levels. Thus, a result of .08% may have the same consequence as a urine test being positive for marijuana. A result of .04% may result in only removal from duty for a period of time. These intermediate results pose some special issues. Let's look at a situation where a person blew .02%. From the employer's standpoint, this individual should not be working. From the employee's perspective, he may have done nothing wrong. He could have taken Nyquil® several hours ago. He could have drunk a lot the night before and claim that he stopped drinking at midnight. Thus, he would not like to be punished when he may not have done anything wrong (i.e., he violated no company policies). The difficulties in using multiple cutoffs do not exist for illicit substances. For drugs like cocaine or marijuana, results are just positive or negative. As a result of trying to regulate an otherwise legal substance like alcohol, we see policies with different thresholds.

The scenario described above where a person has a borderline test from legitimate use outside of work does occur, but not at alarming rates. Many policies prohibit the use of alcohol for a period of time prior to work (such as four hours). The latter situation where someone claims to have been drinking the night before can happen, although it is a little tough. Alcohol metabolizes at different rates in different people. On average, it will metabolize .02% per hour. So, a person who is legally drunk at .08% would have no detectable alcohol in 4 hours. You can see that a person would have to have been drinking pretty heavily the night before to still have detectable levels the next morning. An interesting observation in people who assert the "night before" excuse is that they all claim to have stopped drinking "around midnight." This is true whether I see the person at 7 a.m. or 1 p.m.—"Doc, I was drinking a lot last night but stopped around midnight . . . ." The time has no bearing on the outcome, but I find it interesting.

Lastly, because breath is typically used rather than urine, the testing equipment and testing procedures are conducted differently. Nowadays, saliva testing can be used as an alcohol screen. If it is positive, then the testing center uses breath testing. For our purposes, I will refer to using breath or the combination of saliva and breath as just breath testing. Like urine testing, the testing personnel need to be trained. A chain of custody is still used. The alcohol testing industry has standards for calibrating machines and for ensuring accuracy. Consequently, an acceptable device must be able to distinguish acetone from alcohol. In fact, a device must be listed in the *Federal Register* (A daily publication of the U.S. Government).

Breath alcohol, on the other hand, is accurate for testing purposes. Because it is metabolized fairly quickly, your chance of finding it on pre-employment or random tests is pretty low. More likely than not, testing for alcohol is done based on suspicion. The rapid metabolism of alcohol has an obvious advantage—its detection on breath means that use was recent. Incorporating it into your routine testing is fine and is frequently done because alcohol is the most abused drug in this country. Many employers give employees the option to have blood alcohol tested at the same time as breath (but usually not instead of breath). This is a reasonable practice and gives additional assurance to the breath test. In reality, breath testing by itself is reliable enough.

Interpreting Alcohol Results

Unlike with other drug testing, breath alcohol results are printed when the test is done. Under a DOT program, an MRO is not routinely involved in interpreting results. Since many non-regulated drug testing programs mirror the DOT rules, an MRO does not have a role with most alcohol test results. The result is usually given to an appropriate company representative. Your company can set its own cut-off for a positive result. For convenience, companies frequently use the same level used for legal intoxication. This varies by state, but most use .08% (read as "point zero eight") or .100% ("point one"). Blood test results utilize the same cut-off, but often use different units. So, 80 mg/dl is the same as .08%. In a strict, technical sense, breath test results are not reported as the alcohol level in the breath. Rather, breath levels are proportionate to body levels. The breath machine measures the amount in the breath and performs the calculation so that the result displayed represents that of the body. This is why breath and blood results use the same cut-off level.

A result greater than .08% has the same effect as any other "positive" test. A result of .00% is also straightforward. Anything in between is a little confusing. Remember, in urine drug testing, the report only states negative if the drug level measured is less than the cut-off. In breath testing, it is different. The quantitative result is reported and the employer has to figure out what it means.

OTHER ISSUES

Alternative Tests

I have made a few assumptions in your drug testing program, besides the biggest assumption that you have a program. Firstly, I assume that you are testing urine. There are tests available for hair, fingernail and God knows what else specimens. These are interesting from a technology point of view, but accuracy and interpretation are not standardized. Any conclusions that you make will have some uncertainty and there is not universal agreement about the results. Most significant is that specimens such as hair may indicate *exposure*, rather than *use*. From my standpoint, urine is the way to go. Your goal is not to find drugs at all costs. You need to find a result that is defensible scientifically, medically, and legally.

Another assumption is that after a specimen is collected, it is sent to a laboratory. There are rapid tests available. You can think of them as being similar to rapid pregnancy tests (except the rabbit gets stoned, instead of dying). On the spot, you get a positive or negative answer. Since these are screening tests, a positive result is only preliminary. It must be sent to the lab for confirmation. Reliability is not the issue.

You are left with a problem on your hands if the screen is positive; it is not certain what to do while awaiting a confirmation. Although it can take 2-3 days before the confirmation is back, you have to do something today about the donor. On the one hand, you would not want the person to return to work and then get back a confirmed positive. On the other, you would not want to suspend a person in a punitive fashion and then have the test come back negative. Further, if the confirmation is negative, there is still a potential stigma issue. Some individuals might have a perception that somehow the donor got lucky or some sort of technicality allowed him to beat the test. In the right environment, rapid testing can work well.

Beating the drug test

Adulteration detection is actually a very interesting area of science. It is constantly trying to keep up with methods that people use to thwart drug testing. The basic idea is that the donor tries to get the a drug test to be negative when it should be positive. Often, this is done by adding something to the urine to obscure the testing. Many of these "magic" substances are marketed on the internet or sold in stores. From a law of averages standpoint, I am sure some people are successful. However, the products to thwart a drug test are not as successful as they claim. Suffice it to say that the testing process includes steps to identify when this occurs. Besides using adulteration methods, someone trying to beat a drug test can exploit human behavior. This may include just having someone else provide your specimen. A urine donor can also not sign the chain of custody. Not signing a chain of custody will generally invalidate a test result if the collector did not take note of it. Remember, the collector can document a person's refusal to sign and that would not invalidate a test. These techniques usually include distracting the collection site personnel in some manor so that they do not pick up on these slights of hand. People can also try to beat the test after the results are back. They can claim it was not their test or offer to take a retest. For the most part, testing is good enough to prevent these maneuvers from being effective.

There are always new methods out there to beat the test and the ability to detect them will come about. We have made the process more idiot-proof. Unfortunately, we have made a better idiot.

Releasing Results

It is of obvious importance to determine who can receive test results. Employees may request copies of their actual drug test result. I cannot see why they want it, but it does happen. While your company may not have a particular obligation to provide it, there is probably no reason why you shouldn't. A more difficult situation is when someone else requests it. Other employers or third parties, for example, may want it. Generally, they have no right to it. A common practice is to treat it like other personnel information. That is, many companies won't release it. If a situation came up, you may wish to provide the employee with a copy to allow him/her to do with it what he wants. Companies also worry about whether they have an obligation to notify a third party of positive results. The quick answer is no, but some of the situations where this comes up warrant consulting with legal counsel anyway.

Testing Non-Employees

Some organizations test groups in addition to their own workforce. Most commonly, this would be contractors, students and volunteers. Testing these groups is largely a matter of preference. On the other hand, logistically it is more difficult and some organizations choose not too. I do not have a particular preference other than recommending that if you do this, do it well. You may prefer to have certain non-employees tested, but recognize the additional burden of doing so. One solution is to contract with entities that drug test their own employees. Many temporary agencies do this (it is good for business). In addition to merely asking if they perform drug testing, it is probably worth a casual inquiry about their program. I would ask whether they do just pre-employment or do random as well, what they test for and what happens if someone is positive.

Volunteers are easiest to deal with. They are like employees in many aspects with the exception of not being paid. It makes a lot of sense to test your volunteers if you are testing the rest of the workforce.

Testing students has been a very controversial issues in the context of schools doing it. However, because some education sites are work sites, drug testing students is more plausible in this setting. Additionally, students are often training for jobs where the employed person is being tested (nursing students become nurses). It is challenging for companies to test students who are on their property because the students are transient. The company may not have very good accountability for which students are onsite at a given time. In other words, the group is just too difficult to capture. Other issues present themselves such as training students about your policy and notifying them of a required test. Perhaps the best way to address this is through your agreement with the educational institution. Typically, schools have contracts with education sites. So, informing them that they need to inform their students of the requirement will alleviate some of the burden.

Much of the same logic applies to contractors. The primary rationale for testing contractors is that they perform tasks similar to employees.

Even ones who do other things, but are onsite for an extended period of time, might be tested. Having a computer programmer who is an independent contractor would be an example of someone you might test. Contractors such as someone answering a service call to fix the copier would, therefore, not be tested. It is just too impractical. Trying to test the mail carrier just borders on absurd. Again, you could address the notification issues through your contract with the contracting entity.

CONCLUSION

It should be apparent that developing and maintaining a workplace drug testing program entails work and costs. However, drug testing is becoming increasingly present in today's environment. Most people have probably had experience with drug tests, but many misconceptions still exist. There can never be guarantees of a perfect system. There is not only one way to run a program. Hopefully, I was able to point out some common pitfalls to avoid and was able to discuss common practices.

SAMPLE POLICY

Originally, I intended to provide a sample policy. I then realized this cannot be done. I have seen policies ranging from 3 paragraphs to 20 pages. The information below is not intended to serve as a policy for your organization or any other organization. Rather, it reflects some of the key points noted in other sections of this book. Any organization should consult with their legal counsel and medical advisor before implementing any corporate health policies.

Effective date:

Purpose

Our Company is committed to maintaining a healthy environment, which includes a workplace free from substance abuse. This policy is in compliance with the *Drug Free Workplace Act* [Delete if not pertinent. Other laws or regulations could be listed, if pertinent.] Please direct questions to _____ [List name of responsible individual and how to reach him/her].

Prohibited Conduct

Use of an illicit substance

Unauthorized use of an otherwise legal substance

Use of alcohol while on company premises or while conducting company business

Use of alcohol within 12 hours after an accident or until tested

Presence of a breath test (or blood alcohol) result greater than or equal to .02

Refusal to appear for or submit to a drug testing

Failure to cooperate in the testing process

Unauthorized use of substance includes using medication prescribed to a different individual. It also includes using medication obtained in a different country if its use or possession in the United States is prohibited. An employee who wishes to use a medication obtained in another country should have the substance prescribed by his/her physician in the United States to substantiate appropriate use. Unauthorized use includes using medication prescribed to the employee, but used in a manner inconsistent with how it is prescribed.

Definitions

Drug Testing

Our Company conducts drug testing in the following circumstances:
Pre-employment / Pre-hire—Testing occurring before the first day of work. All employees are tested prior working. Job offers are contingent on passing a urine drug test. [Many organizations have trainees, students, consultants, and contractors who are not employees, but they wish to test. Include all pertinent categories.]

Random—Unannounced testing. All persons in designated safety sensitive positions are subject to random testing.

List of safety sensitive positions
1.
2.

Post-accident—Any accident or incident occurring while on Our Company premises, while operating a Our Company vehicle or conducting Our Company business where there is a death or injury cost estimate of greater than $500 or property damage cost estimate greater than $500.

For Cause / Reasonable Suspicion—Testing as a result of an employee demonstrating behavior or conduct consistent with substance abuse. All employees are subject to For Cause testing.

Follow up Testing—Testing that occurs after an employee has returned to work following prohibited conduct due to substance abuse. It also includes when such an employee is initially returning to work.

All urine drug testing shall be conducted by a laboratory certified by the United States Department of Health and Human services. Breath alcohol testing is conducted by a facility having proficiency in alcohol testing.

Procedures for Testing

Human resources schedules job candidates for their pre-employment test. Human resources must contact the job candidate at least 24 hours prior to the test and provide appropriate instructions. The Supervisor, Human Resources is responsible for selecting employees for random testing. Randomly selected employees should be notified no more than 2 hours prior to their test. Employees who are not properly notified are not subject to the "refusal to test" provisions of this policy. Employees who are scheduled off when selected do not need to be notified and are not expected to be tested. If testing an employee would be substantially disruptive to the operations of Our Company, then he/she can be excluded from testing. However, the determination that testing is substantially disruptive is the responsibility of the Supervisor, Human Resources. Managers or the selected employee who believe that providing a specimen would be substantially disruptive must discuss the situation with the Supervisor, Human Resources immediately.

Employees must sign-in at the collection site at their designated appointment time or within two hours of notification for random testing. Failure to do so is considered a "refusal to test." Likewise, an employee who does not provide an adequate specimen while at collection site is subject to "refusal to test" provisions. An employee who has an appropriate medical explanation for not providing a specimen is not subject to the "refusal to test" provisions. The medical review officer determines whether there was an appropriate medical explanation.

Test Results

All urine drug test results from the laboratory are reviewed by the Medical Review Officer. The MRO determines the final result as "positive", "negative", or other appropriate confirmed result.

Results of pre hire tests are maintained as long as other material, forms, and applications used in the application and hiring process. Results of other tests are maintained in drug test files maintained by human resources. These files are confidential and separate from other personnel file material and are separate from medical files. [State laws and agency regulations may set their own retention rules.]

A negative result has no adverse personnel action. A positive result requires a person be removed from duty. In addition, a person is subject to termination. As an alternative, a person is offered an opportunity to seek appropriate rehabilitation. Rehabilitation costs are the responsibility of the employee, although insurance may cover certain costs. A person seeking to return to work after rehabilitation must seek clearance though ____ and will be required to sign a return to work agreement.

A refusal to test or adulterating or attempting to adulterate a urine drug screen can result in immediate termination.